The Art of Ear Reflexology

A Compendium of Techniques and Applications

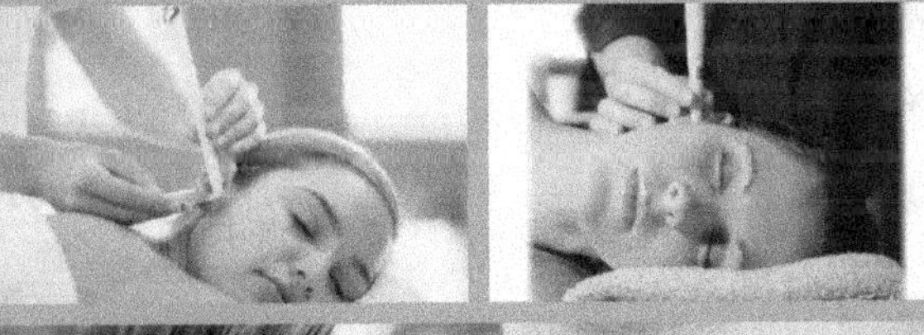

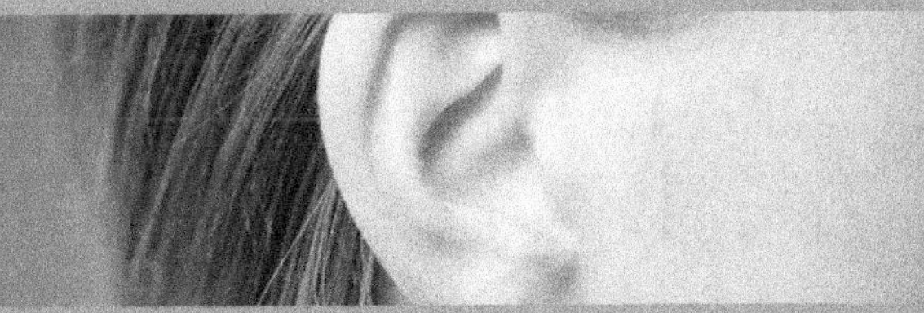

Dr. James K. Ferguson

COPYRIGHT © 2024 by Dr.

James K. Ferguson

All rights reserved. No part of this publication may be reproduced, distributed, or transmitted in any form or by any means, including photocopying, recording, or other electronic or mechanical methods, without the prior written permission of the copyright owner, except in the case of brief quotations embodied in critical reviews and certain other noncommercial uses permitted by copyright law.

TABLE OF CONTENTS

INTRODUCTION

Welcome to the world of ear reflexology, where the ears are not just for hearing but also for healing. In this comprehensive compendium , you will embark on a journey of discovery into the ancient art of auricular therapy, exploring how the stimulation of specific points on the ear can promote health and well-being throughout the body.

What is Ear Reflexology?: Ear reflexology, also known as auriculotherapy, is based on the principle that the ear is a microsystem of the entire body, with each part of the ear corresponding to a specific organ or function. By stimulating these points through massage, pressure, or other techniques, it is believed that one can alleviate pain, reduce stress, and improve overall health.

History and Origins: The practice of ear reflexology can be traced back to ancient Egypt, China, and Greece, where healers and physicians used ear manipulation to treat various ailments. In modern times, the technique was further developed by French physician Dr. Paul Nogier in the 1950s, who mapped out the ear into specific reflex zones.

Benefits of Ear Reflexology: Ear reflexology offers a range of benefits for both physical and mental health. It is known to promote relaxation, reduce stress and anxiety, improve circulation, relieve pain, and enhance overall well-being. Many people also find that ear reflexology helps them sleep better and improves their mood.

How Does Ear Reflexology Differ from Foot or Hand Reflexology?: While foot and hand reflexology focus on specific reflex points on the feet and hands, ear reflexology targets points on the outer ear. The ear is believed to be particularly sensitive to reflexology because it is richly supplied with nerves and has a close connection to the brain.

Your Journey with Ear Reflexology: In this compendium , you will learn everything you need to know to practice ear reflexology effectively. From understanding the anatomy of the ear to mastering the techniques and exploring the reflex points, each chapter will guide you step-by-step through the process.

As you delve into the world of ear reflexology, keep an open mind and a curious spirit. The techniques you will learn in this compendium have the potential to transform not just your health but your entire outlook on life. So, let us embark on this journey together, as we discover the healing power of the ears.

CHAPTER 1

20 important things you should know about Ear Reflexology

1. Ear reflexology, also known as auricular therapy, is a holistic therapy that involves stimulating specific points on the ear to promote healing and relaxation in corresponding areas of the body.

2. Ear reflexology is based on the principle that the ear is a microsystem of the body, with each part of the ear corresponding to a different organ or body part.

3. This therapy is believed to help improve circulation, reduce tension, and promote overall well-being.

4. Ear reflexology can be used to address a wide range of health issues, including pain, stress, insomnia, and digestive problems.

5. Ear reflexology is a non-invasive therapy that is generally safe for most people, although it may not be suitable for those with certain ear conditions or medical issues.

6. A session of ear reflexology typically lasts between 15 and 30 minutes and can be a relaxing and rejuvenating experience.

7. Regular ear reflexology sessions may help improve overall health and well-being by promoting relaxation and reducing stress.

8. Ear reflexology is suitable for people of all ages, from children to the elderly.

9. It is important to choose a qualified and experienced reflexologist when seeking ear reflexology treatment.

10. Ear reflexology is not a substitute for medical care, and it is important to consult with a healthcare professional for any serious health concerns.

11. Some people may experience discomfort during an ear reflexology session, but this is usually temporary and should subside quickly.

12. Ear reflexology can be a beneficial therapy for those looking to improve their overall health and well-being in a natural and holistic way.

13. The practice of ear reflexology has been used for thousands of years in various cultures around the world.

14. Ear reflexology is believed to help balance the body's energy and promote a sense of harmony and well-being.

15. Some research suggests that ear reflexology may be effective in reducing pain and improving quality of life for people with certain health conditions.

16. Ear reflexology can be a cost-effective and non-invasive way to improve your health and well-being.

17. Many people find that ear reflexology helps them feel more relaxed and rejuvenated, with improved ear health and function.

18. Ear reflexology can be easily incorporated into your daily self-care routine for added benefits.

19. Overall, ear reflexology is a safe and effective therapy that can help improve your health and well-being in a natural and holistic way.

20. Learning and practicing ear reflexology can be a rewarding experience, providing you with valuable self-care tools for life.

CHAPTER 2

Overview of Ear Reflexology

Ear reflexology, also known as auricular therapy, is a holistic healing technique that involves stimulating specific points on the ear to promote health and well-being in various parts of the body. It is based on the principle that the outer ear is a microsystem that reflects the entire body, similar to how the feet and hands are mapped in foot and hand reflexology.

The practice of ear reflexology dates back to ancient times, with records indicating its use in ancient Egypt, China, and Greece. In modern times, the technique was further developed by French physician Dr. Paul Nogier in the 1950s, who mapped out the ear into specific reflex zones.

The ear is divided into several zones, each corresponding to a different part of the body. By stimulating these zones through massage, pressure, or other techniques, it is believed that one can alleviate pain, reduce stress, and improve overall health.

Ear reflexology is often used as a complementary therapy to conventional medical treatments. It is non-invasive and generally safe when practiced by a trained professional. Many people find it to be a relaxing and enjoyable experience, and it is often used to promote relaxation and reduce stress.

Research on the effectiveness of ear reflexology is ongoing, with some studies suggesting that it may be beneficial for certain conditions such as pain management, anxiety, and insomnia. However, more research is needed to fully understand its potential benefits and mechanisms of action.

History and Origins of Ear Reflexology

The practice of using the ear as a map to treat ailments and promote healing dates back thousands of years. Ancient cultures such as the Egyptians, Chinese, and Greeks all recognized the therapeutic properties of the ear. In ancient Egypt, for example, hieroglyphics depict medical practitioners using ear cones to treat various conditions.

The modern practice of ear reflexology, however, is largely attributed to the work of Dr. Paul Nogier, a French physician, in the 1950s. Dr. Nogier observed that the ear could be mapped to correspond to different parts of the body, much like the feet and hands in reflexology. He developed the concept of the "homunculus" on the ear, where the ear is seen as a microcosm of the body, with each part of the ear corresponding to a specific body part or organ.

Dr. Nogier's work laid the foundation for modern ear reflexology, and his maps and theories are still used by practitioners today. Since then, ear reflexology has gained popularity as a complementary therapy to promote relaxation, reduce stress, and alleviate various ailments.

Today, ear reflexology is practiced worldwide and is often used alongside other holistic therapies to promote overall health and well-being. Its long history and continued use are a testament to its effectiveness and enduring appeal.

Benefits of Ear Reflexology

Ear reflexology offers a myriad of potential benefits for both physical and mental well-being. **Here are some key benefits:**

1. Stress Reduction: Stimulating the reflex points on the ear can help to relax the body and mind, reducing stress and promoting a sense of calmness.

2. Pain Relief: Ear reflexology is believed to help alleviate various types of pain, including headaches, migraines, and joint pain.

3. Improved Circulation: By stimulating the ear reflex points, blood flow to different parts of the body may be improved, which can help with overall circulation.

4. Enhanced Relaxation and Sleep: Many people find that ear reflexology helps them to relax deeply, which can improve sleep quality and overall well-being.

5. Balancing Energy Flow: According to traditional Chinese medicine, stimulating the ear reflex points can help to balance the flow of energy, or Qi, in the body, promoting health and vitality.

6. Support for the Immune System: Some practitioners believe that ear reflexology can help to strengthen the immune system, making the body more resilient to illness and disease.

7. Digestive Support: Ear reflexology is thought to help improve digestion and relieve symptoms of digestive disorders such as bloating, indigestion, and constipation.

8. Mental Clarity and Focus: Stimulating certain ear reflex points may help to improve mental clarity, focus, and concentration.

9. Emotional Balance: Ear reflexology is believed to help balance emotions, reduce anxiety, and promote a sense of well-being.

10. Complementary Therapy: Ear reflexology can be used alongside conventional medical treatments to support overall health and well-being.

It's important to note that while many people find ear reflexology to be beneficial, individual results may vary. It's always a good idea to consult with a qualified healthcare professional before starting any new therapy or treatment.

How Ear Reflexology Differs from Foot or Hand Reflexology

Ear reflexology, foot reflexology, and hand reflexology are all based on the principle that specific points on these areas correspond to different organs and systems in the body. While they share this fundamental concept, there are several key differences between them:

1. Location of Reflex Points: In ear reflexology, the reflex points are located on the outer ear, which is believed to mirror the entire body. In foot reflexology, the reflex points are located on the feet, and in hand reflexology, they are located on the hands.

2. Size of Reflex Area: The ear is a relatively small area compared to the feet and hands, which means that the reflex points on the ear are more densely packed. This can make it easier to target specific points in ear reflexology.

3. Accessibility: The feet and hands are more accessible for self-massage and reflexology techniques, making foot and hand reflexology more practical for self-care. Ear reflexology often requires the assistance of a trained practitioner.

4. Sensitivity of Reflex Points: Some people find that the reflex points on the ears are more sensitive than those on the feet or hands, which can affect the way they respond to reflexology techniques.

5. Application of Pressure: The pressure applied during ear reflexology is typically gentler compared to foot reflexology, as the ear is a delicate and sensitive area.

6. Integration with Traditional Chinese Medicine: In traditional Chinese medicine, the ears are considered a microsystem that reflects the entire body, making ear reflexology an integral part of TCM healing practices.

Despite these differences, all three forms of reflexology are believed to promote relaxation, reduce stress, and support overall health and well-being. Each individual may respond differently to each type of reflexology, so it's important to explore and find what works best for you.

CHAPTER 3

Understanding Ear Reflexology

Ear reflexology, also known as auricular therapy, is a holistic healing practice that involves stimulating specific points on the outer ear to promote health and well-being in the body. This therapy is based on the belief that the ear is a microsystem that reflects the entire body, similar to how the feet and hands are mapped in foot and hand reflexology.

The concept of ear reflexology is rooted in traditional Chinese medicine, where the ear is seen as a complex map of the body's organs, systems, and functions. According to this theory, each part of the ear corresponds to a specific area of the body, and by stimulating these points, one can help to restore balance and harmony to the body's energy flow.

Ear reflexology is often used as a complementary therapy to conventional medical treatments. It is non-invasive and generally safe when practiced by a trained professional. Many people find it to be a relaxing and enjoyable experience, and it is often used to promote relaxation, reduce stress, and alleviate various ailments.

Practitioners of ear reflexology use various techniques to stimulate the reflex points on the ear, including massage, acupressure, and the use of small seeds or pellets that are taped to specific points on the ear and left in place for a period of time.

Research on the effectiveness of ear reflexology is ongoing, with some studies suggesting that it may be beneficial for conditions such as pain management, anxiety, and insomnia. However, more research is needed to fully understand its potential benefits and mechanisms of action.

Overall, ear reflexology is a gentle and natural therapy that can be used to promote health and well-being in a holistic manner. Whether used alone or in combination with other therapies, it offers a unique and effective way to support the body's natural healing processes.

Anatomy of the Ear: A Guide to Understanding Ear Reflexology

To understand how ear reflexology works, it's essential to first understand the anatomy of the ear. The ear is a complex and intricate organ responsible for hearing and balance. It is divided into three main parts: the outer ear, the middle ear, and the inner ear.

1. Outer Ear: The outer ear consists of the pinna (also known as the auricle) and the ear canal. The pinna is the visible part of the ear that collects sound waves and directs them into the ear canal. The ear canal is a tube-like structure that leads to the eardrum.

2. Middle Ear: The middle ear is a small, air-filled cavity located behind the eardrum. It contains three small bones called the ossicles (the malleus, incus, and stapes) that transmit sound vibrations from the eardrum to the inner ear.

3. Inner Ear: The inner ear is a complex structure located deep within the skull. It contains the cochlea, which is responsible for hearing, and the vestibular system, which is responsible for balance. The cochlea is a spiral-shaped organ filled with fluid and tiny hair cells that convert sound vibrations into electrical signals that are sent to the brain. The vestibular system consists of three semicircular canals that detect changes in head position and movement.

In ear reflexology, the outer ear is the focus of attention, as it is believed to contain reflex points that correspond to different parts of the body. These reflex points are thought to be connected to the body's energy pathways, or meridians, and stimulating them is believed to help restore balance and promote healing.

By understanding the anatomy of the ear and the location of its reflex points, practitioners of ear reflexology can target specific areas of the body and provide targeted therapy to promote health and well-being.

Mapping the Ear for Reflexology: Understanding Auricular Therapy

Ear reflexology, also known as auricular therapy, is based on the principle that specific points on the ear correspond to different parts of the body. The ear is divided into several zones or maps, each of which is believed to represent a different part of the body. By stimulating these points, practitioners aim to promote healing and balance in the corresponding body parts.

One of the most commonly used maps in ear reflexology is the inverted fetus map. In this map, the ear is believed to resemble an inverted fetus, with the head located at the lower part of the earlobe and the feet at the top of the ear near the helix. The body's organs and systems are thought to be represented along the curved ridge of the ear, with specific points corresponding to specific areas of the body.

Another important map in ear reflexology is the somatotopic map, which divides the ear into zones that correspond to specific body parts. For example, the earlobe is believed to correspond to the head and neck, while the upper part of the ear corresponds to the lower body.

In addition to these maps, there are also points on the ear that are believed to have specific functions, such as the Shen Men point, which is thought to promote relaxation and reduce stress, and the Thalamus point, which is believed to help with pain relief.

Practitioners of ear reflexology use these maps and points to guide their treatment. By stimulating the appropriate points on the ear, they aim to restore balance and harmony to the body's energy flow, promoting health and well-being.

Principles of Ear Reflexology: Understanding the Basis of Auricular Therapy

Ear reflexology, or auricular therapy, is based on several key principles that guide its practice and effectiveness. These principles are rooted in traditional Chinese medicine and the concept of the ear as a microsystem that reflects the entire body.

Here are the fundamental principles of ear reflexology:

1. Holistic Approach: Ear reflexology takes a holistic approach to health and wellness, viewing the body as an interconnected system where imbalances in one part can affect the whole. By stimulating specific points on the ear, practitioners aim to restore balance and harmony to the body as a whole.

2. Energy Flow: Central to the principles of ear reflexology is the concept of energy flow, or Qi (pronounced "chee"), within the body. It is believed that disruptions or blockages in the flow of Qi can lead to illness and disease. By stimulating the reflex points on the ear, practitioners aim to unblock stagnant energy and promote the free flow of Qi throughout the body.

3. Microsystem Theory: The ear is seen as a microsystem that reflects the entire body. This means that specific points on the ear correspond to specific organs, systems, and functions in the body. By stimulating these points, practitioners can affect change in the corresponding areas of the body.

4. Natural Healing: Ear reflexology is based on the belief that the body has an innate ability to heal itself. By stimulating the reflex points on the ear, practitioners aim to activate the body's natural healing mechanisms and promote self-healing.

5. Complementary Therapy: Ear reflexology is often used as a complementary therapy to conventional medical treatments. It is non-invasive and generally safe, making it a popular choice for those looking for natural and holistic approaches to health and wellness.

Overall, the principles of ear reflexology emphasize the interconnectedness of the body, mind, and spirit, and the importance of addressing imbalances at a holistic level to promote health and well-being.

CHAPTER 4

Techniques of Ear Reflexology: Exploring Auricular Therapy Methods

Ear reflexology employs several techniques to stimulate specific points on the ear to promote health and well-being. These techniques are based on the principle that the ear is a microsystem that reflects the entire body, and by stimulating these points, practitioners aim to restore balance and harmony to the body's energy flow.

Here are some common techniques used in ear reflexology:

1. Massage: Massaging the ear with gentle pressure is one of the most common techniques used in ear reflexology. Practitioners use their fingers to massage and knead the earlobe, the outer edges of the ear, and the curved ridge of the ear to stimulate the reflex points.

2. Acupressure: Acupressure involves applying pressure to specific points on the ear using the fingers or a small tool. This pressure is believed to help unblock stagnant energy and promote the free flow of Qi throughout the body.

3. Ear Seeds: Ear seeds are small, adhesive seeds or pellets that are placed on specific points on the ear and left in place for a period of time. These seeds apply constant pressure to the reflex points, stimulating them and promoting healing.

4. Ear Reflexology Tools: Specialized tools, such as ear reflexology probes or rollers, may be used to stimulate the reflex points on the ear. These tools are designed to apply gentle pressure and massage to the ear, promoting relaxation and healing.

5. Ear Candles: Some practitioners use ear candles, hollow cones made of fabric soaked in beeswax or paraffin, to stimulate the ear reflex points. The heat and smoke from the ear candle are believed to help draw out impurities and promote healing.

6. Auricular Taping: Auricular taping involves using tape to secure small magnets or seeds to specific points on the ear. This technique provides continuous stimulation to the reflex points and can be used as a form of self-care between sessions with a practitioner.

7.   Electrostimulation: In some cases, electrostimulation may be used to stimulate the reflex points on the ear. This technique involves applying a mild electrical current to the ear, which is believed to help restore balance to the body's energy flow.

Overall, the techniques of ear reflexology are gentle, non-invasive, and generally safe when practiced by a trained professional. They can be used alone or in combination with other holistic therapies to promote health and well-being.

Preparation and Tools Needed for Ear Reflexology

Preparing for an ear reflexology session involves creating a calm and comfortable environment to promote relaxation and healing.

Here are some steps to prepare for an ear reflexology session, along with the tools needed:

1. Prepare the Environment: Find a quiet and comfortable space where you can relax undisturbed. Dim the lights, play soft music if desired, and ensure the room is at a comfortable temperature.

2. Gather Supplies: Collect the tools and supplies you will need for the session, including ear seeds or pellets, massage oil or lotion, cotton swabs, and a mirror if necessary.

3. Clean the Ear: Use a gentle cleanser to clean the outer ear and remove any dirt or debris. This will ensure that the reflex points are easily accessible and that the treatment is effective.

4. Positioning: Sit or lie down in a comfortable position with your head supported. This will help you relax and allow the practitioner to access the ear reflex points easily.

5. Techniques and Tools: The tools needed for ear reflexology include your hands for massage, ear seeds or pellets for acupressure, and possibly ear candles or other specialized tools. These tools are used to stimulate the reflex points on the ear and promote healing.

6. Massage Oil or Lotion: Some practitioners use massage oil or lotion to help lubricate the ear and make the massage more comfortable. Choose a natural, unscented oil or lotion for the best results.

7. Cotton Swabs: Cotton swabs can be used to apply pressure to specific points on the ear or to remove excess oil or lotion after the session.

8. Mirror: A mirror may be used to help locate specific points on the ear, especially for self-care techniques.

9. Comfortable Clothing: Wear loose, comfortable clothing that allows easy access to the ears for the session.

10. Relaxation Techniques: Practice deep breathing or other relaxation techniques to help you relax and prepare for the session.

By preparing the environment and gathering the necessary tools and supplies, you can ensure that your ear reflexology session is effective and enjoyable, promoting relaxation and healing.

Basic Ear Reflexology Techniques: Simple Methods for Self-Care

Ear reflexology can be a simple and effective way to promote relaxation and well-being.

Here are some basic techniques that you can use for self-care:

1. Ear Massage: Gently massage the outer ear with your thumb and forefinger, using small circular motions. Start at the earlobe and work your way up to the top of the ear. This can help to stimulate the reflex points and promote relaxation.

2. Ear Pulling: Gently pull on the earlobe and outer edges of the ear, using a gentle, rhythmic motion. This can help to stimulate the reflex points and improve circulation in the ear.

3. Acupressure: Use your thumb or a small tool to apply gentle pressure to specific points on the ear. You can find these points by referring to a ear reflexology chart. Hold the pressure for a few seconds, then release. Repeat this process for each point you want to stimulate.

4. Ear Seeds: Place a small ear seed or pellet on a specific point on the ear and secure it with adhesive tape. Leave the seed in place for several hours or overnight to stimulate the reflex point.

5. Auricular Taping: Use adhesive tape to secure small magnets or seeds to specific points on the ear. This provides continuous stimulation to the reflex points and can be used for self-care between sessions with a practitioner.

6. Ear Candle Treatment: This technique involves using a hollow cone-shaped candle that is placed in the ear and lit at the other end. The heat and smoke from the candle are believed to help draw out impurities and promote healing. This technique should only be done by a trained professional.

7. Warm Compress: Applying a warm compress to the ear can help to relax the muscles and improve circulation. This can be especially helpful for relieving tension and promoting relaxation.

These basic ear reflexology techniques can be easily incorporated into your daily routine for self-care. They are safe and gentle, but if you have any specific health concerns or conditions, it's always best to consult with a healthcare professional before trying any new therapy.

Advanced Techniques and Variations in Ear Reflexology

While basic ear reflexology techniques can be effective for general relaxation and well-being, there are also advanced techniques and variations that can be used to target specific issues or provide a more tailored treatment.

Here are some advanced techniques and variations in ear reflexology:

1. In-Depth Point Stimulation: Instead of just massaging or applying pressure to the ear reflex points, practitioners may use more specific and detailed techniques to target each point. This can include using different levels of pressure, varying the speed and direction of the strokes, and incorporating other techniques such as kneading or tapping.

2. Zone Therapy: Zone therapy involves dividing the ear into zones that correspond to different parts of the body, similar to the somatotopic map used in foot reflexology. By focusing on specific zones, practitioners can provide a more targeted treatment that addresses specific health issues or concerns.

3. Integration with Traditional Chinese Medicine (TCM): In TCM, the ear is seen as a microsystem that reflects the entire body. Practitioners may incorporate TCM principles and techniques into their ear reflexology practice, such as using specific acupoints or meridians to address imbalances in the body's energy flow.

4. Auricular Acupuncture: Some practitioners may combine ear reflexology with auricular acupuncture, which involves inserting small needles into specific points on the ear to stimulate the reflex points. This can provide a more intense and targeted treatment for certain conditions.

5. Auricular Aromatherapy: Aromatherapy can be incorporated into ear reflexology by using essential oils that are applied to the ear or inhaled during the treatment. This can enhance the therapeutic effects of the treatment and promote relaxation and healing.

6. Ear Reflexology Tools: Specialized tools, such as ear reflexology probes or rollers, may be used to stimulate the reflex points on the ear. These tools can provide a more precise and targeted treatment, especially for hard-to-reach or sensitive areas of the ear.

7. Combination Therapies: Ear reflexology can be combined with other holistic therapies, such as foot reflexology, hand reflexology, or massage therapy, to provide a more comprehensive treatment that addresses the body as a whole.

Overall, advanced techniques and variations in ear reflexology can provide a more personalized and effective treatment that addresses specific health issues or concerns. Practitioners may use a combination of these techniques to create a treatment plan that is tailored to each individual's needs.

CHAPTER 5

Reflexology Points on the Ear: Understanding the Key Points for Healing

Ear reflexology involves stimulating specific points on the ear that are believed to correspond to different parts of the body. These reflex points are thought to be connected to the body's energy pathways, or meridians, and stimulating them is believed to help restore balance and promote healing.

Here are some of the key reflexology points on the ear:

1. Auricle: The auricle, or outer part of the ear, is divided into zones that correspond to different parts of the body. The earlobe corresponds to the head and neck, the upper part of the ear corresponds to the upper body, and the lower part of the ear corresponds to the lower body.

2. Shen Men: Located in the upper part of the ear, the Shen Men point is believed to promote relaxation, reduce stress, and relieve pain. It is often used as a general tonic for overall health and well-being.

3. Kidney Point: Located at the bottom of the earlobe, the kidney point is believed to correspond to the kidneys and urinary system. Stimulating this point is thought to help improve kidney function and promote detoxification.

4. Liver Point: Located on the lower edge of the ear, the liver point is believed to correspond to the liver and gallbladder. Stimulating this point is thought to help improve liver function and promote detoxification.

5. Spleen Point: Located on the upper edge of the ear, the spleen point is believed to correspond to the spleen and digestive system. Stimulating this point is thought to help improve digestion and boost the immune system.

6. Lung Point: Located in the middle of the ear, the lung point is believed to correspond to the lungs and respiratory system. Stimulating this point is thought to help improve lung function and promote respiratory health.

7. Heart Point: Located in the upper part of the ear, the heart point is believed to correspond to the heart and cardiovascular system. Stimulating this point is thought to help improve heart health and circulation.

8. Endocrine Points: There are several points on the ear that are believed to correspond to the endocrine glands, including the pituitary, thyroid, and adrenal glands. Stimulating these points is thought to help balance hormone levels and promote overall hormonal health.

By stimulating these reflexology points on the ear, practitioners aim to promote relaxation, reduce stress, and support overall health and well-being. Each point may be stimulated using various techniques, such as massage, acupressure, or ear seeds, depending on the individual's needs and preferences.

Major Reflex Points on the Ear and Their Corresponding Areas

Ear reflexology involves stimulating specific points on the ear that are believed to correspond to different parts of the body.

Here are some major reflex points on the ear and their corresponding areas:

1. Brain: Located on the upper part of the ear, near the top of the ear canal. Stimulating this point is believed to help improve brain function and mental clarity.

2. Eyes: Located on the upper outer edge of the ear. Stimulating this point is believed to help improve vision and eye health.

3. Nose and Sinuses: Located on the inner upper edge of the ear. Stimulating this point is believed to help relieve sinus congestion and improve respiratory health.

4. Mouth and Throat: Located on the lower outer edge of the ear. Stimulating this point is believed to help improve oral health and throat conditions.

5. Heart: Located in the upper central part of the ear. Stimulating this point is believed to help improve heart health and circulation.

6. Lungs: Located in the middle part of the ear. Stimulating this point is believed to help improve lung function and respiratory health.

7. Liver: Located on the lower edge of the ear. Stimulating this point is believed to help improve liver function and detoxification.

8. Kidneys: Located at the bottom of the earlobe. Stimulating this point is believed to help improve kidney function and detoxification.

9. Digestive System: Located on the inner lower edge of the ear. Stimulating this point is believed to help improve digestion and relieve digestive issues.

10. Endocrine System: There are several points on the ear that correspond to the endocrine glands, including the pituitary, thyroid, and adrenal glands. Stimulating these points is believed to help balance hormone levels and promote overall hormonal health.

By stimulating these major reflex points on the ear, practitioners aim to promote balance and harmony in the corresponding areas of the body, leading to improved health and well-being.

Lesser-Known Reflex Points on the Ear and Their Benefits

In addition to the major reflex points on the ear, there are also lesser-known reflex points that are believed to have specific benefits when stimulated.

Here are some of these lesser-known reflex points and their benefits:

1. Shoulder and Neck: Located at the top of the ear, near the outer edge. Stimulating this point is believed to help relieve tension and stiffness in the shoulders and neck.

2. Elbow: Located on the upper outer edge of the ear, near the top. Stimulating this point is believed to help relieve pain and discomfort in the elbows.

3. Wrist: Located on the upper inner edge of the ear, near the top. Stimulating this point is believed to help improve circulation and relieve wrist pain.

4. Hip: Located on the lower outer edge of the ear, near the bottom. Stimulating this point is believed to help relieve hip pain and improve hip mobility.

5. Knee: Located on the lower inner edge of the ear, near the bottom. Stimulating this point is believed to help relieve knee pain and improve knee function.

6. Ankle: Located on the lower outer edge of the ear, near the bottom. Stimulating this point is believed to help relieve ankle pain and improve ankle mobility.

7. Feet: Located on the lower inner edge of the ear, near the bottom. Stimulating this point is believed to help improve circulation and relieve foot pain.

8. Emotional Points: There are several points on the ear that are believed to correspond to emotions, such as anxiety, stress, and sadness.

Stimulating these points is believed to help promote emotional balance and well-being.

By stimulating these lesser-known reflex points on the ear, practitioners aim to provide targeted relief for specific issues and promote overall balance and harmony in the body.

CHAPTER 6

Ear Reflexology for Common Ailments: Using Auricular Therapy for Relief

Ear reflexology, also known as auricular therapy, can be used to help alleviate a variety of common ailments and promote overall health and well-being.

Here are some common ailments that ear reflexology can help with:

1. Headaches and Migraines: Stimulating the reflex points on the ear that correspond to the head and neck can help to relieve tension and reduce the frequency and intensity of headaches and migraines.

2. Stress and Anxiety: Ear reflexology is believed to help promote relaxation and reduce stress and anxiety. Stimulating the reflex points on the ear can help to calm the mind and promote a sense of well-being.

3. Insomnia and Sleep Disorders: Stimulating the reflex points on the ear that correspond to the brain and nervous system can help to promote relaxation and improve sleep quality.

4. Digestive Issues: Ear reflexology can help to improve digestion and relieve symptoms of digestive disorders such as bloating, indigestion, and constipation. Stimulating the reflex points on the ear that correspond to the digestive system can help to promote better digestion.

5. Pain Relief: Ear reflexology can help to relieve various types of pain, including joint pain, back pain, and muscle pain. Stimulating the reflex points on the ear that correspond to the affected area can help to reduce pain and promote healing.

6. Immune System Support: Ear reflexology is believed to help strengthen the immune system and make the body more resilient to illness and disease. Stimulating the reflex points on the ear that correspond to the immune system can help to boost immunity.

7. Menstrual Cramps: Stimulating the reflex points on the ear that correspond to the reproductive system can help to relieve menstrual cramps and promote hormonal balance.

8. Respiratory Issues: Ear reflexology can help to improve respiratory health and relieve symptoms of respiratory conditions such as asthma and bronchitis. Stimulating the reflex points on the ear that correspond to the lungs and respiratory system can help to promote better breathing.

By using ear reflexology for these common ailments, you can help to alleviate symptoms and promote overall health and well-being. It's important to note that while ear reflexology can be a helpful complementary therapy, it should not be used as a substitute for conventional medical treatment. If you have a serious or chronic health condition, it's always best to consult with a healthcare professional before trying any new therapy.

Ear Reflexology for Stress and Anxiety Relief: Calming the Mind and Body

Stress and anxiety are common issues that can have a significant impact on our overall health and well-being. Ear reflexology, also known as auricular therapy, can be a powerful tool for relieving stress and anxiety and promoting relaxation.

Here's how ear reflexology can help:

1. Shen Men Point: The Shen Men point is located in the upper part of the ear and is often referred to as the "heavenly gate." Stimulating this point is believed to promote relaxation, reduce stress, and calm the mind.

2. Adrenal Point: The adrenal point is located on the lower inner edge of the ear, near the bottom. Stimulating this point is believed to help regulate the body's stress response and promote a sense of calm.

3. Sympathetic Nervous System: The ear is rich in nerve endings that are connected to the sympathetic nervous system, which is responsible for the body's "fight or flight" response to stress. Stimulating these nerve endings can help to calm the sympathetic nervous system and promote relaxation.

4. Endorphin Release: Stimulating the reflex points on the ear can trigger the release of endorphins, which are the body's natural "feel-good" chemicals. This can help to reduce pain and promote a sense of well-being.

5. Overall Relaxation: Ear reflexology is a relaxing and soothing treatment that can help to calm the mind and body. The gentle pressure and massage techniques used in ear reflexology can help to promote relaxation and reduce tension.

To use ear reflexology for stress and anxiety relief, you can gently massage the reflex points on the ear using your thumb and forefinger, or use ear seeds or pellets to apply gentle pressure to the points. It's important to find a quiet and comfortable space where you can relax undisturbed during the treatment. With regular practice, ear reflexology can be a valuable tool for managing stress and anxiety and promoting overall health and well-being.

Ear Reflexology for Pain Management: Alleviating Discomfort Naturally

Ear reflexology can be an effective natural therapy for managing various types of pain. By stimulating specific reflex points on the ear, you can help alleviate pain and promote healing. **Here's how ear reflexology can help with pain management:**

1. Endorphin Release: Stimulating the reflex points on the ear can trigger the release of endorphins, which are the body's natural painkillers. This can help to reduce pain and promote a sense of well-being.

2. Gate Control Theory: According to the gate control theory of pain, stimulating nerve endings in one area of the body can help to block pain signals from reaching the brain. By stimulating the reflex points on the ear, you can help to block pain signals and reduce discomfort.

3. Relaxation Response: Ear reflexology is a relaxing and soothing therapy that can help to calm the mind and body. This can be especially helpful for managing pain that is exacerbated by stress or tension.

4. Specific Reflex Points: There are specific reflex points on the ear that are believed to correspond to different parts of the body. By stimulating these points, you can help alleviate pain in specific areas. For example, stimulating the shoulder and neck reflex points on the ear can help relieve tension headaches and neck pain.

5. Complementary Therapy: Ear reflexology can be used as a complementary therapy alongside conventional pain management techniques. It can help to enhance the effectiveness of other treatments and reduce the need for pain medication.

To use ear reflexology for pain management, you can gently massage the reflex points on the ear using your thumb and forefinger, or use ear seeds or pellets to apply gentle pressure to the points. It's important to communicate with your healthcare provider before using ear reflexology for pain management, especially if you have a chronic or severe pain condition.

Ear Reflexology for Digestive Disorders: Promoting Digestive Health Naturally

Ear reflexology can be a gentle and effective natural therapy for managing digestive disorders and promoting overall digestive health. By stimulating specific reflex points on the ear, you can help alleviate digestive issues and support optimal digestion.

Here's how ear reflexology can help with digestive disorders:

1. Stimulation of Digestive Reflex Points: There are specific reflex points on the ear that are believed to correspond to the digestive system, including the stomach, intestines, and liver. By stimulating these points, you can help to improve digestion and relieve symptoms of digestive disorders.

2. Relaxation Response: Ear reflexology is a relaxing therapy that can help to calm the mind and body. This can be especially helpful for managing digestive issues that are exacerbated by stress or tension.

3. Improved Circulation: Stimulating the reflex points on the ear can help to improve circulation to the digestive organs, which can promote better digestion and nutrient absorption.

4. Detoxification: Ear reflexology is believed to help promote detoxification and elimination of waste from the body. This can help to relieve symptoms of bloating, gas, and constipation.

5. Complementary Therapy: Ear reflexology can be used as a complementary therapy alongside other treatments for digestive disorders, such as dietary changes and medications. It can help to enhance the effectiveness of these treatments and promote overall digestive health.

To use ear reflexology for digestive disorders, you can gently massage the reflex points on the ear using your thumb and forefinger, or use ear seeds or pellets to apply gentle pressure to the points. It's important to communicate with your healthcare provider before using ear reflexology for digestive disorders, especially if you have a chronic or severe digestive condition.

Ear Reflexology for Insomnia and Sleep Disorders: Enhancing Sleep Quality Naturally

Ear reflexology can be a beneficial natural therapy for improving sleep quality and managing insomnia and other sleep disorders. By stimulating specific reflex points on the ear, you can help promote relaxation, reduce stress, and improve overall sleep patterns.

Here's how ear reflexology can help with insomnia and sleep disorders:

1. Stress Reduction: Ear reflexology is believed to help reduce stress and promote relaxation, which can be beneficial for improving sleep quality. By stimulating the reflex points on the ear, you can help calm the mind and body, making it easier to fall asleep.

2. Endorphin Release: Stimulating the reflex points on the ear can trigger the release of endorphins, which are the body's natural "feel-good" chemicals. This can help to promote a sense of well-being and relaxation, which can aid in falling asleep and staying asleep.

3. Regulation of Circadian Rhythms: Ear reflexology is thought to help regulate the body's internal clock, or circadian rhythms, which play a crucial role in determining sleep patterns. By stimulating the reflex points on the ear, you can help reset your body's natural sleep-wake cycle.

4. Relief from Restless Legs Syndrome (RLS): Ear reflexology can also help alleviate symptoms of restless legs syndrome, a common sleep disorder characterized by uncomfortable sensations in the legs and an uncontrollable urge to move them. Stimulating specific reflex points on the ear can help reduce these symptoms and improve sleep quality.

5. Complementary Therapy: Ear reflexology can be used as a complementary therapy alongside other treatments for insomnia and sleep disorders, such as cognitive behavioral therapy for insomnia (CBT-I) or medications. It can help enhance the effectiveness of these treatments and promote better sleep.

To use ear reflexology for insomnia and sleep disorders, you can gently massage the reflex points on the ear using your thumb and forefinger, or use ear seeds or pellets to apply gentle pressure to the points. It's important to communicate with your healthcare provider before using ear reflexology for sleep issues, especially if you have a chronic or severe sleep disorder.

Ear Reflexology for Respiratory Issues: Supporting Respiratory Health Naturally

Ear reflexology can be a beneficial natural therapy for managing respiratory issues and promoting overall respiratory health. By stimulating specific reflex points on the ear, you can help alleviate symptoms of respiratory conditions such as asthma, bronchitis, and allergies.

Here's how ear reflexology can help with respiratory issues:

1. Lung Point Stimulation: Stimulating the reflex points on the ear that correspond to the lungs and respiratory system can help improve lung function and promote clearer breathing. This can be especially beneficial for managing symptoms of asthma and bronchitis.

2. Sinus Relief: Ear reflexology can help relieve sinus congestion and promote clearer sinuses. Stimulating the reflex points on the ear that correspond to the sinuses can help reduce symptoms of sinusitis and allergies.

3. Immune System Support: Ear reflexology is believed to help strengthen the immune system, making the body more resilient to respiratory infections. Stimulating the reflex points on the ear that correspond to the immune system can help boost immunity.

4. Relaxation Response: Ear reflexology is a relaxing therapy that can help reduce stress and tension, which can be beneficial for managing respiratory issues that are exacerbated by stress.

5. Complementary Therapy: Ear reflexology can be used as a complementary therapy alongside other treatments for respiratory issues, such as medication and breathing exercises. It can help enhance the effectiveness of these treatments and promote overall respiratory health.

To use ear reflexology for respiratory issues, you can gently massage the reflex points on the ear using your thumb and forefinger, or use ear seeds or pellets to apply gentle pressure to the points. It's important to communicate with your healthcare provider before using ear reflexology for respiratory issues, especially if you have a chronic or severe respiratory condition.

Ear Reflexology for Menstrual and Hormonal Imbalances: Supporting Women's Health Naturally

Ear reflexology can be a beneficial natural therapy for managing menstrual and hormonal imbalances in women. By stimulating specific reflex points on the ear, you can help alleviate symptoms of PMS (premenstrual syndrome), menstrual cramps, and hormonal imbalances. **Here's how ear reflexology can help with menstrual and hormonal issues:**

1. Hormonal Balance: Stimulating the reflex points on the ear that correspond to the endocrine glands, such as the pituitary, thyroid, and adrenal glands, can help balance hormone levels and promote overall hormonal health.

2. Menstrual Cramp Relief: Ear reflexology can help relieve menstrual cramps by stimulating the reflex points on the ear that correspond to the reproductive organs. This can help reduce pain and discomfort associated with menstruation.

3. PMS Symptoms: Ear reflexology can help alleviate symptoms of PMS, such as mood swings, bloating, and fatigue. Stimulating the reflex points on the ear can help balance mood and energy levels, making it easier to cope with PMS symptoms.

4. Regulation of Menstrual Cycle: Ear reflexology is believed to help regulate the menstrual cycle by balancing hormone levels and promoting optimal reproductive health.

5. Stress Reduction: Ear reflexology is a relaxing therapy that can help reduce stress and tension, which can be beneficial for managing menstrual and hormonal issues that are exacerbated by stress.

6. Complementary Therapy: Ear reflexology can be used as a complementary therapy alongside other treatments for menstrual and hormonal imbalances, such as dietary changes and hormone therapy. It can help enhance the effectiveness of these treatments and promote overall women's health.

To use ear reflexology for menstrual and hormonal imbalances, you can gently massage the reflex points on the ear using your thumb and forefinger, or use ear seeds or pellets to apply gentle pressure to the points. It's important to communicate with your healthcare provider before using ear reflexology for menstrual and hormonal issues, especially if you have a chronic or severe condition.

CHAPTER 7

Incorporating Ear Reflexology Into Your Life: Simple Steps for Wellness

Ear reflexology can be a valuable tool for promoting wellness and balance in your life. By incorporating ear reflexology into your daily routine, you can help support your overall health and well-being.

Here are some simple steps for incorporating ear reflexology into your life:

1. Self-Massage: Take a few minutes each day to gently massage the reflex points on your ears. Use your thumb and forefinger to apply gentle pressure to the points, starting with the earlobe and working your way up to the top of the ear. This can help promote relaxation and reduce stress.

2. Ear Seeds or Pellets: Consider using ear seeds or pellets to apply gentle pressure to the reflex points on your ears throughout the day. These small, adhesive seeds can be placed on the reflex points and left in place for several hours to provide continuous stimulation.

3. Relaxation Technique: Use ear reflexology as a relaxation technique whenever you feel stressed or tense. Take a few minutes to gently massage your ears or apply pressure to the reflex points to help calm your mind and body.

4. Bedtime Routine: Incorporate ear reflexology into your bedtime routine to help promote better sleep. Gently massage your ears before bed to help relax your body and mind, making it easier to fall asleep.

5. Complement to Other Therapies: Use ear reflexology as a complement to other wellness therapies, such as massage, acupuncture, or aromatherapy. By combining these therapies, you can enhance their effectiveness and promote overall wellness.

6. Consult a Professional: If you're new to ear reflexology or have specific health concerns, consider consulting a professional reflexologist. They can provide guidance on how to incorporate ear reflexology into your life and tailor a treatment plan to meet your individual needs.

Incorporating ear reflexology into your life can be a simple and effective way to support your overall health and well-being. Whether you use it as a relaxation technique, a complement to other therapies, or as part of your daily routine, ear reflexology can help promote wellness and balance in your life.

Self-Administered Ear Reflexology Techniques: Promoting Wellness at Home

Ear reflexology can be a simple and effective way to promote wellness and balance in your life. By learning some self-administered ear reflexology techniques, you can easily incorporate this practice into your daily routine. **Here are some techniques you can try at home:**

1. Ear Massage: Gently massage your ears using your thumb and forefinger. Start at the earlobe and work your way up to the top of the ear, using circular motions. This can help promote relaxation and reduce stress.

2. Ear Pulling: Gently pull on your earlobes and the outer edges of your ears. This can help stimulate the reflex points on your ears and promote circulation.

3. Ear Rolling: Roll the outer edges of your ears between your thumb and forefinger. This can help stimulate the reflex points on your ears and promote relaxation.

4. Ear Pressing: Use your thumb to apply gentle pressure to the reflex points on your ears. Hold the pressure for a few seconds, then release. Repeat this process for each reflex point on your ears.

5. Ear Seeds or Pellets: Apply ear seeds or pellets to the reflex points on your ears. These small, adhesive seeds can be left in place for several hours to provide continuous stimulation.

6. Auricular Acupressure: Use your thumb to apply pressure to specific acupressure points on your ears. These points are believed to correspond to different parts of the body and can help promote overall wellness.

7. Deep Breathing: While stimulating the reflex points on your ears, practice deep breathing. This can help enhance the relaxation response and promote overall well-being.

8. Mindfulness Meditation: Practice mindfulness meditation while stimulating the reflex points on your ears. This can help calm your mind and reduce stress.

By incorporating these self-administered ear reflexology techniques into your daily routine, you can promote wellness and balance in your life. Experiment with different techniques to find what works best for you, and enjoy the benefits of ear reflexology at home.

Integrating Ear Reflexology into Your Daily Routine: Simple Steps for Wellness

Integrating ear reflexology into your daily routine can be a powerful way to promote wellness and balance in your life. By incorporating ear reflexology into your daily activities, you can easily reap the benefits of this practice.

Here are some simple steps for integrating ear reflexology into your daily routine:

1. Morning Routine: Start your day with a few minutes of ear reflexology. Gently massage your ears or apply pressure to the reflex points to help wake up your body and mind.

2. Midday Break: Take a short break during the day to practice ear reflexology. This can help relieve stress and tension, and improve your focus and productivity.

3. Evening Relaxation: Wind down in the evening with a relaxing ear reflexology session.

This can help calm your mind and body, making it easier to unwind and prepare for sleep.

4. Complement to Other Activities: Integrate ear reflexology into other wellness activities, such as yoga or meditation. Practice ear reflexology while practicing these activities to enhance their benefits.

5. Mindful Moments: Use ear reflexology as a mindfulness practice. Take a few moments throughout the day to practice ear reflexology mindfully, focusing on the sensations in your ears and the relaxation it brings.

6. Incorporate into Self-Care Routine: Include ear reflexology as part of your self-care routine. This can help you feel more balanced and grounded, and improve your overall well-being.

7. Experiment with Techniques: Explore different ear reflexology techniques to find what works best for you. Try massaging, pressing, or using ear seeds to stimulate the reflex points on your ears.

8. Set Intentions: Before practicing ear reflexology, set an intention for your practice. Whether it's to reduce stress, improve digestion, or enhance relaxation, setting an intention can help focus your practice and maximize its benefits.

By integrating ear reflexology into your daily routine, you can promote wellness and balance in your life. Experiment with different techniques and find what works best for you, and enjoy the benefits of ear reflexology as part of your daily life.

Safety Precautions and Contraindications for Ear Reflexology

While ear reflexology is generally safe for most people, there are some precautions and contraindications to be aware of. It's important to consult with a healthcare professional before starting any new wellness practice, especially if you have any underlying health conditions.

Here are some safety precautions and contraindications for ear reflexology:

1. Pregnancy: If you are pregnant, consult with your healthcare provider before practicing ear reflexology. Some reflex points on the ear are believed to correspond to reproductive organs, and stimulation of these points could potentially affect pregnancy.

2. Infections or Injuries: Avoid practicing ear reflexology on areas of the ear that are infected or injured. This could worsen the condition or cause further complications.

3. Skin Conditions: If you have any skin conditions on or around your ears, such as eczema or psoriasis, be gentle when practicing ear reflexology to avoid irritating the skin further.

4. Allergies: Be cautious if you have allergies to adhesive materials, as some ear reflexology techniques involve using ear seeds or pellets that adhere to the skin.

5. Medical Conditions: If you have any medical conditions, such as epilepsy or a heart condition, consult with your healthcare provider before practicing ear reflexology, as it may not be suitable for you.

6. Medications: If you are taking any medications, especially blood thinners, consult with your healthcare provider before practicing ear reflexology, as it may interact with your medication.

7. Professional Guidance: If you are new to car reflexology, consider seeking guidance from a professional reflexologist to ensure you are using the correct techniques and applying the right amount of pressure.

8. Discontinue if Uncomfortable: If you experience any discomfort or pain during ear reflexology, discontinue the practice and consult with a healthcare professional.

By following these safety precautions and contraindications, you can practice ear reflexology safely and effectively. Listen to your body and consult with a healthcare professional if you have any concerns.

CHAPTER 8

Ear Reflexology for Special Populations: Tailoring Techniques for Different Needs

Ear reflexology can be adapted to suit the needs of special populations, including children, the elderly, and individuals with specific health conditions. By tailoring techniques to meet the needs of these populations, you can help promote wellness and balance in a safe and effective way.

Here are some considerations for practicing ear reflexology with special populations:

1. Children: When practicing ear reflexology with children, use gentle and soothing techniques. Children may have smaller ears and be more sensitive to pressure, so be mindful of this when applying pressure to the reflex points. Keep the sessions short and engaging to hold their attention.

2. Elderly: With the elderly, use gentle and slow techniques, as their skin may be more fragile. Be mindful of any medical conditions they may have, such as arthritis or diabetes, and adapt your techniques accordingly. Keep the sessions short and comfortable for them.

3. Pregnant Women: When practicing ear reflexology with pregnant women, avoid stimulating reflex points that are believed to correspond to reproductive organs. Focus instead on points that promote relaxation and stress relief. Always consult with their healthcare provider before starting any new wellness practice.

4. Individuals with Chronic Conditions: For individuals with chronic conditions such as diabetes, hypertension, or arthritis, be cautious when applying pressure to the reflex points. Consult with their healthcare provider before starting ear reflexology to ensure it is safe for them.

5. Individuals with Disabilities: For individuals with disabilities, adapt your techniques to suit their needs. Use gentle and soothing techniques, and be mindful of their comfort level. Consider using ear seeds or pellets as an alternative to manual pressure.

6. End-of-Life Care: For individuals receiving end-of-life care, ear reflexology can be a gentle and comforting practice. Use gentle and soothing techniques to promote relaxation and reduce pain and discomfort.

7. Professional Guidance: When working with special populations, consider seeking guidance from a professional reflexologist who has experience working with these populations. They can provide guidance on techniques and adaptations to ensure a safe and effective practice.

By tailoring ear reflexology techniques to meet the needs of special populations, you can help promote wellness and balance in a gentle and effective way. Listen to the individual's needs and adapt your techniques accordingly, always keeping their safety and comfort in mind.

Ear Reflexology for Children: Gentle Techniques for Wellness

Ear reflexology can be a gentle and effective way to promote wellness in children. By using gentle techniques and adapting the practice to suit their needs, you can help support their overall health and well-being.

Here are some tips for practicing ear reflexology with children:

1. Use Gentle Pressure: Children's ears are more delicate than adults', so use gentle pressure when practicing ear reflexology. Use your thumb and forefinger to apply light pressure to the reflex points on their ears.

2. Keep Sessions Short and Engaging: Children may have shorter attention spans, so keep ear reflexology sessions short and engaging. Make it fun by incorporating games or storytelling into the session.

3. Focus on Relaxation: Ear reflexology can help children relax and reduce stress. Focus on using techniques that promote relaxation, such as gentle massage and light pressure.

4. Tailor Techniques to Their Needs: Children may have different needs than adults, so tailor your techniques to suit their needs. For example, if a child is experiencing digestive issues, focus on the reflex points on the ear that correspond to the digestive system.

5. Be Mindful of Their Comfort: Pay attention to the child's comfort level during the session. If they are uncomfortable or in pain, stop the session immediately.

6. Use Ear Seeds or Pellets: Ear seeds or pellets can be a gentle alternative to manual pressure for children. These small, adhesive seeds can be placed on the reflex points on their ears and left in place for several hours to provide continuous stimulation.

7. Consult with a Healthcare Professional: If you have any concerns about practicing ear reflexology with your child, consult with a healthcare professional. They can provide guidance on techniques and safety precautions.

By practicing ear reflexology with children in a gentle and mindful way, you can help promote their overall health and well-being. Listen to their needs and adapt your techniques to suit them, always keeping their comfort and safety in mind.

Ear Reflexology for the Elderly: Gentle Techniques for Comfort and Wellness

Ear reflexology can be a gentle and soothing practice for the elderly, promoting relaxation and overall well-being. When working with elderly individuals, it's important to use gentle techniques and adapt the practice to suit their needs.

Here are some tips for practicing ear reflexology with the elderly:

1. Gentle Pressure: Use gentle pressure when practicing ear reflexology with the elderly. Their skin may be more fragile, so it's important to be gentle to avoid causing discomfort or injury.

2. Slow and Relaxing Techniques: Use slow and relaxing techniques to promote relaxation. Gentle massage and light pressure can help soothe tension and promote a sense of calm.

3. Focus on Comfort: Pay attention to the elderly person's comfort level during the session. If they experience any discomfort, adjust your techniques accordingly or stop the session if necessary.

4. Adapt to Their Needs: The elderly may have specific health concerns or conditions that require special attention. Adapt your techniques to suit their needs, focusing on areas that may benefit their health, such as reflex points related to circulation or digestion.

5. Shorter Sessions: Keep ear reflexology sessions short and comfortable for the elderly. They may not be able to tolerate longer sessions, so it's important to be mindful of their comfort.

6. Consult with Healthcare Providers: If the elderly person has any underlying health conditions or concerns, consult with their healthcare provider before practicing ear reflexology. They can provide guidance on techniques and safety precautions.

7. Use Ear Seeds or Pellets: Ear seeds or pellets can be a gentle alternative to manual pressure for the elderly. These small, adhesive seeds can be placed on the reflex points on their ears and left in place for several hours to provide continuous stimulation.

By practicing ear reflexology with the elderly in a gentle and mindful way, you can help promote their comfort and well-being. Listen to their needs and adapt your techniques to suit them, always keeping their comfort and safety in mind.

Ear Reflexology in Pregnancy: Safe Practices for Maternal Wellness

Ear reflexology can be a gentle and effective practice for promoting wellness during pregnancy. However, it's important to use caution and consult with a healthcare provider before practicing ear reflexology during pregnancy, especially in the first trimester.

Here are some safe practices for using ear reflexology during pregnancy:

1. Consult with a Healthcare Provider: Before practicing ear reflexology during pregnancy, consult with your healthcare provider. They can provide guidance on safe techniques and ensure that ear reflexology is appropriate for you.

2. Gentle Techniques: Use gentle techniques when practicing ear reflexology during pregnancy. Avoid applying firm pressure to the reflex points on the ear, especially those believed to correspond to reproductive organs.

3. Focus on Relaxation: Use ear reflexology techniques that promote relaxation and stress relief. This can help alleviate common pregnancy discomforts and promote a sense of well-being.

4. Avoid Certain Reflex Points: Some reflex points on the ear are believed to correspond to reproductive organs. Avoid stimulating these points during pregnancy to avoid potential complications.

5. Short Sessions: Keep ear reflexology sessions short and comfortable for pregnant women. They may not be able to tolerate longer sessions, so it's important to be mindful of their comfort.

6. Hydrate: Pregnant women should stay hydrated before and after ear reflexology sessions to help flush out toxins and support overall wellness.

7. Listen to Your Body: If you experience any discomfort or pain during an ear reflexology session, stop immediately and consult with your healthcare provider.

By practicing ear reflexology safely during pregnancy, you can help promote relaxation and wellness. However, it's important to use caution and consult with a healthcare provider to ensure that ear reflexology is safe for you and your baby.

CHAPTER 9

Complementary Practices to Enhance Ear Reflexology

Ear reflexology can be complemented by various practices to enhance its benefits and promote overall well-being. By combining ear reflexology with other complementary practices, you can create a holistic approach to wellness. **Here are some complementary practices that can enhance the effects of ear reflexology:**

1. Aromatherapy: Use essential oils to enhance the relaxation and therapeutic effects of ear reflexology. Apply a drop of diluted essential oil to your fingertips before massaging the reflex points on your ears, or use a diffuser to fill the room with calming scents.

2. Breathing Exercises: Practice deep breathing exercises while stimulating the reflex points on your ears. Deep breathing can help promote relaxation and reduce stress, enhancing the effects of ear reflexology.

3. Meditation: Incorporate meditation into your ear reflexology practice to promote mental clarity and relaxation. Focus on your breath and the sensations in your ears as you stimulate the reflex points.

4. Yoga: Practice gentle yoga poses that focus on relaxation and stress relief before or after ear reflexology. Yoga can help release tension in the body and enhance the effects of ear reflexology.

5. Acupressure: Combine ear reflexology with acupressure techniques to stimulate specific points on the body. Acupressure can help balance the body's energy and enhance the effects of ear reflexology.

6. Massage: Receive a full-body massage before or after ear reflexology to promote relaxation and circulation. Massage can help prepare the body for ear reflexology and enhance its effects.

7. Herbal Remedies: Use herbal remedies, such as teas or tinctures, to support your wellness goals alongside ear reflexology. Consult with a healthcare provider or herbalist to find the right herbs for your needs.

8. Mindfulness Practices: Practice mindfulness throughout your day to enhance the effects of ear reflexology. Be present and aware of your body and surroundings, allowing yourself to fully experience the benefits of ear reflexology.

By incorporating these complementary practices into your ear reflexology routine, you can enhance its benefits and promote overall well-being. Experiment with different practices to find what works best for you, and enjoy the holistic approach to wellness that ear reflexology offers.

Acupressure and Acupuncture: Traditional Therapies for Wellness

Acupressure and acupuncture are traditional Chinese therapies that have been used for centuries to promote wellness and treat various health conditions. While acupressure involves applying pressure to specific points on the body, acupuncture uses fine needles to stimulate these points. Both therapies are based on the concept of qi (pronounced "chee"), or life force energy, which flows through the body along pathways called meridians.

Acupressure: Acupressure is a gentle and non-invasive therapy that can be easily incorporated into your daily routine. By applying pressure to specific points on the body, you can help balance the flow of qi and promote overall wellness.

Here are some key points about acupressure:

Pressure Points: Acupressure points are located along the body's meridians, which are specific pathways where qi flows. By applying pressure to these points, you can help restore the balance of qi and alleviate symptoms of various health conditions.

Techniques: Acupressure techniques vary depending on the point being stimulated. Common techniques include using the fingers, palms, or elbows to apply pressure to the point in a circular or tapping motion.

Benefits: Acupressure can help promote relaxation, reduce stress, alleviate pain, improve digestion, and support overall well-being. It can be used as a standalone therapy or combined with other treatments for enhanced benefits.

Safety: Acupressure is generally safe when practiced correctly. However, it's important to avoid applying pressure to certain points during pregnancy or if you have a specific health condition. Consult with a qualified acupressure practitioner before starting treatment.

Acupuncture: Acupuncture is a form of traditional Chinese medicine that involves inserting fine needles into specific points on the body to stimulate the flow of qi and restore balance.

Here are some key points about acupuncture:

Needles: Acupuncture needles are very thin and are inserted into the skin at specific depths depending on the point being targeted. The needles are sterile and disposable, ensuring safety and cleanliness.

Meridians: Acupuncture points are located along the body's meridians, which correspond to specific organs and functions of the body. By stimulating these points, acupuncturists can help restore balance and promote healing.

Benefits: Acupuncture is used to treat a wide range of health conditions, including chronic pain, digestive disorders, respiratory issues, and emotional imbalances. It can also help promote relaxation and reduce stress.

Safety: Acupuncture is generally safe when performed by a qualified and licensed acupuncturist. The needles used are very thin and cause minimal discomfort. However, it's important to inform your acupuncturist of any health conditions or medications you are taking before treatment.

Both acupressure and acupuncture are holistic therapies that can help promote wellness and balance in the body. By stimulating specific points on the body, these therapies can help support your body's natural healing process and improve your overall health and well-being.

Aromatherapy: Using Essential Oils for Wellness

Aromatherapy is a holistic therapy that uses essential oils to promote health and well-being. Essential oils are concentrated plant extracts that capture the natural aroma and beneficial properties of plants. When inhaled or applied to the skin, these oils can have a variety of therapeutic effects on the body and mind.

Here's an overview of aromatherapy and how it can be used for wellness:

How Aromatherapy Works:

Inhalation: The most common way to use essential oils in aromatherapy is through inhalation. When you inhale the aroma of essential oils, the molecules travel to the olfactory system, which is connected to the brain. This can trigger various physiological and emotional responses.

Absorption: Essential oils can also be absorbed through the skin. When applied topically, the oils are absorbed into the bloodstream and can have localized or systemic effects on the body.

Benefits of Aromatherapy:

Relaxation and Stress Relief: Many essential oils have calming and relaxing properties, making them ideal for reducing stress and anxiety. Oils such as lavender, chamomile, and bergamot are commonly used for this purpose.

Improved Sleep: Certain essential oils, such as lavender and chamomile, are known for their sedative properties and can help promote better sleep.

Pain Relief: Some essential oils, such as peppermint and eucalyptus, have analgesic properties and can help alleviate pain and inflammation.

Mood Enhancement: Aromatherapy can help uplift the mood and improve mental clarity. Oils such as lemon, orange, and rosemary are known for their invigorating effects.

How to Use Aromatherapy: Diffusion: Use an essential oil diffuser to disperse the aroma of the oil into the air. This is a simple and effective way to enjoy the benefits of aromatherapy.

Massage: Dilute essential oils in a carrier oil, such as jojoba or coconut oil, and use them for massage. This can help relax the muscles and improve circulation.

Bath: Add a few drops of essential oil to a warm bath to create a soothing and relaxing experience.

Inhalation: Place a few drops of essential oil on a tissue or cloth and inhale deeply.

Skin Care: Use essential oils in your skincare routine by adding a few drops to your moisturizer or face mask.

Safety Considerations:

Dilution: Essential oils are highly concentrated and should be diluted before applying to the skin to avoid irritation or sensitization. Use a carrier oil, such as jojoba or coconut oil, to dilute the essential oil.

Patch Test: Perform a patch test before using a new essential oil to check for any allergic reactions or sensitivities.

Pregnancy: Some essential oils should be avoided during pregnancy, so it's important to consult with a healthcare provider before using aromatherapy.

Aromatherapy is a versatile and effective holistic therapy that can be used to promote wellness in various ways. Whether you're looking to relax, improve your mood, or alleviate pain, there's an essential oil that can help support your health and well-being.

Herbal Remedies: Harnessing Nature's Healing Power

Herbal remedies have been used for centuries to promote health and treat various ailments. These natural remedies are derived from plants and herbs and can be used in various forms, including teas, tinctures, capsules, and extracts. **Here's an overview of herbal remedies and how they can be used to support wellness:**

Benefits of Herbal Remedies:

Natural Healing: Herbal remedies work with the body's natural healing processes to promote wellness and balance. They often have fewer side effects than conventional medications.

Holistic Approach: Herbal remedies take a holistic approach to health, addressing the underlying causes of illness rather than just treating symptoms.

Affordability: Herbal remedies are often more affordable than prescription medications, making them accessible to a wide range of people.

Variety of Uses: Herbal remedies can be used to treat a wide range of health conditions, including digestive issues, respiratory problems, skin conditions, and more.

Common Herbal Remedies

Echinacea: Echinacea is often used to boost the immune system and prevent colds and flu.

Ginger: Ginger is known for its anti-inflammatory properties and is often used to treat digestive issues such as nausea and indigestion.

Chamomile: Chamomile is known for its calming properties and is often used to promote relaxation and improve sleep.

St. John's Wort: St. John's Wort is used to treat mild to moderate depression and anxiety.

Peppermint: Peppermint is often used to relieve digestive issues such as gas, bloating, and indigestion.

How to Use Herbal Remedies

Teas: Herbal teas are a popular way to consume herbal remedies. Simply steep the herbs in hot water for several minutes, then strain and drink.

Tinctures: Tinctures are liquid extracts of herbs that are usually taken orally. They are highly concentrated and should be used according to the manufacturer's instructions.

Capsules: Herbal remedies are also available in capsule form, which can be convenient for those who prefer a more standardized dose.

Topical Applications: Some herbal remedies can be applied topically to the skin to treat various skin conditions or relieve pain and inflammation.

Safety Considerations:

Quality: When using herbal remedies, it's important to use high-quality herbs from reputable sources to ensure their safety and effectiveness.

Dosage: Follow the recommended dosage instructions for herbal remedies. Taking too much can be harmful.

Interactions: Some herbal remedies can interact with medications or other herbs, so it's important to consult with a healthcare provider before using herbal remedies, especially if you are taking medications.

Herbal remedies can be a safe and effective way to support your health and well-being. By incorporating these natural remedies into your routine, you can take a proactive approach to your health and enjoy the benefits of nature's healing power.

Massage Techniques: Enhancing Relaxation and Wellness

Massage is a therapeutic technique that involves the manipulation of soft tissues in the body to promote relaxation, relieve tension, and improve circulation. There are many different types of massage techniques, each with its own benefits and uses.

Here are some common massage techniques and their benefits:

Swedish Massage:

Technique: Swedish massage involves long, gliding strokes, kneading, and circular movements on the superficial layers of muscles.

Benefits: It can help relax the entire body, improve circulation, and reduce stress and tension.

Deep Tissue Massage:

Technique: Deep tissue massage targets the deeper layers of muscles and connective tissue using slow, deep strokes and firm pressure.

Benefits: It can help relieve chronic muscle tension, improve range of motion, and reduce inflammation.

Sports Massage:

Technique: Sports massage is specifically designed for athletes and involves a combination of techniques to help prevent injuries, prepare the body for athletic activity, and aid in recovery after exertion.

Benefits: It can help improve athletic performance, reduce muscle soreness, and prevent injuries.

Hot Stone Massage:

Technique: Hot stone massage involves the use of heated stones placed on specific parts of the body to help relax muscles and improve circulation. The therapist may also use the stones to massage the body.

Benefits: It can help promote relaxation, relieve muscle tension, and improve circulation.

Aromatherapy Massage:

Technique: Aromatherapy massage combines massage techniques with the use of essential oils to enhance the therapeutic effects of the massage.

Benefits: It can help promote relaxation, reduce stress and anxiety, and improve mood.

Thai Massage:

Technique: Thai massage involves a combination of acupressure, stretching, and assisted yoga postures. The therapist uses their hands, knees, legs, and feet to move you into a series of yoga-like stretches.

Benefits: It can help improve flexibility, relieve muscle and joint tension, and promote overall relaxation.

Shiatsu Massage:

Technique: Shiatsu massage is a form of Japanese bodywork that involves applying pressure to specific points on the body using the fingers, thumbs, and palms.

Benefits: It can help promote relaxation, relieve stress and tension, and improve circulation.

Benefits of Massage

Relaxation: Massage can help relax the body and mind, reducing stress and promoting a sense of well-being.

Pain Relief: Massage can help relieve muscle tension, reduce pain, and improve flexibility and range of motion.

Improved Circulation: Massage can help improve blood circulation, which can promote healing and reduce swelling.

Enhanced Mood: Massage can help release endorphins, which are natural mood enhancers, leading to a better sense of well-being.

Safety Considerations:

Medical Conditions: If you have any medical conditions or concerns, consult with your healthcare provider before receiving a massage.

Pregnancy: If you are pregnant, consult with your healthcare provider before receiving a massage, as some techniques may not be suitable during pregnancy.

Allergies: If you have any allergies, inform your massage therapist before the session, especially if aromatherapy oils are being used.

Comfort: Communicate with your massage therapist about your comfort level during the session, including pressure, temperature, and areas of focus.

CHAPTER 10

Case Studies and Success Stories In Massage Therapy

Massage therapy has been shown to have numerous benefits for both physical and mental health.

Here are some case studies and success stories that highlight the positive effects of massage therapy:

Case Study 1: Chronic Pain Relief

Patient Profile: A 45-year-old woman with chronic lower back pain.

Treatment: The patient received weekly deep tissue massages focusing on the lower back area.

Results: After six weeks of treatment, the patient reported a significant reduction in pain and an improvement in mobility. She was able to resume daily activities without discomfort.

Case Study 2: Stress and Anxiety Reduction

Patient Profile: A 30-year-old man experiencing high levels of stress and anxiety.

Treatment: The patient received weekly Swedish massages focusing on relaxation techniques.

Results: After four weeks of treatment, the patient reported feeling more relaxed and less anxious. He also experienced improved sleep quality and overall mood.

Case Study 3: Sports Injury Recovery

Patient Profile: A 25-year-old athlete recovering from a hamstring injury.

Treatment: The patient received bi-weekly sports massages focusing on the injured area.

Results: After six weeks of treatment, the patient reported a significant improvement in flexibility and reduced pain. He was able to return to training sooner than expected.

Success Story 1: Migraine Relief

Patient: A 35-year-old woman suffering from frequent migraines.

Treatment: The patient received monthly massages focusing on the neck and shoulder area.

Results: After three months of treatment, the patient reported a decrease in the frequency and severity of migraines. She also experienced improved posture and reduced muscle tension.

Success Story 2: Postpartum Depression

Patient: A 28-year-old woman experiencing postpartum depression.

Treatment: The patient received bi-weekly massages focusing on relaxation and stress relief.

Results: After six weeks of treatment, the patient reported feeling more positive and less overwhelmed. She also experienced improved sleep and bonding with her baby.

Success Story 3: Fibromyalgia Management

Patient: A 50-year-old woman diagnosed with fibromyalgia.

Treatment: The patient received weekly massages focusing on pain relief and muscle relaxation.

Results: After three months of treatment, the patient reported a significant reduction in pain and fatigue. She also experienced improved sleep quality and overall well-being.

These case studies and success stories demonstrate the positive impact that massage therapy can have on various health conditions. From chronic pain relief to stress reduction, massage therapy offers a holistic approach to wellness that can benefit individuals of all ages and backgrounds.

Real-Life Experiences with Ear Reflexology

Ear reflexology, also known as auriculotherapy, has gained popularity as a natural therapy for promoting relaxation and wellness.

Here are some real-life experiences of individuals who have tried ear reflexology:

Case Study 1: Stress Relief

Name: Sarah

Age: 35

Occupation: Office Manager

Experience: Sarah had been experiencing high levels of stress due to her demanding job. She decided to try ear reflexology as a natural way to relax. After a few sessions, Sarah noticed a significant reduction in her stress levels. She felt more calm and balanced, and her sleep improved. Sarah continues to incorporate ear reflexology into her routine as a way to manage stress.

Case Study 2: Pain Management

Name: Mark

Age: 50

Occupation: Construction Worker

Experience: Mark had been suffering from chronic back pain for years due to his job. He tried various treatments with limited success. A friend recommended ear reflexology, and Mark decided to give it a try. After several sessions, Mark noticed a reduction in his back pain. He felt more comfortable and was able to move more freely. Mark continues to receive regular ear reflexology treatments to manage his pain.

Case Study 3: Improved Sleep

Name: Emily

Age: 42

Occupation: Teacher

Experience: Emily had been struggling with insomnia for months, which was affecting her work and daily life. She tried ear reflexology as a natural remedy for her sleep issues. After a few sessions, Emily noticed that she was able to fall asleep faster and stay asleep longer. She felt more rested and alert during the day. Emily now uses ear reflexology as part of her bedtime routine to promote better sleep.

Case Study 4: Digestive Health

Name: David

Age: 55

Occupation: Retired

Experience: David had been dealing with digestive issues, including bloating and indigestion, for years. He tried various medications with limited success. A friend suggested ear reflexology as a natural remedy for his digestive problems. After a few sessions, David noticed an improvement in his digestion. His symptoms became less frequent, and he felt more comfortable after meals. David continues to use ear reflexology to support his digestive health.

These real-life experiences highlight the potential benefits of ear reflexology for promoting relaxation, managing pain, improving sleep, and supporting digestive health. While individual experiences may vary, many people find ear reflexology to be a gentle and effective therapy for enhancing their overall well-being.

Testimonials and Feedback on Ear Reflexology

Here are some testimonials and feedback from individuals who have experienced ear reflexology:

1. Jennifer, 40: "I have been struggling with anxiety for years, and ear reflexology has been a game-changer for me. It helps me relax and calm my mind, and I feel more balanced after each session."

2. Michael, 55: "I started receiving ear reflexology treatments for my chronic neck pain, and I am amazed at the results. My pain has significantly reduced, and I feel more comfortable in my daily activities."

3. Sara, 30: "I was skeptical about ear reflexology at first, but after trying it, I am a believer. It has helped me manage my stress levels and improve my overall well-being. I highly recommend it to anyone looking for a natural way to relax."

4. John, 45: "I have been dealing with digestive issues for years, and ear reflexology has been a lifesaver for me. It has helped me reduce bloating and improve my digestion. I feel much better after each session."

5. Emma, 50: "I have been using ear reflexology to help me sleep better, and it has worked wonders. I fall asleep faster and stay asleep longer, and I wake up feeling more refreshed and energized."

6. David, 35: "I have tried various therapies for my back pain, but nothing has worked as well as ear reflexology. It has helped me manage my pain and improve my mobility. I am so grateful for this treatment."

These testimonials highlight the positive experiences that individuals have had with ear reflexology. Many people find it to be a gentle and effective therapy for promoting relaxation, managing pain, improving sleep, and supporting overall well-being.

CHAPTER 11

Questions and Answers About Ear Reflexology

1. What is ear reflexology?

Ear reflexology, also known as auriculotherapy, is a form of alternative medicine that involves applying pressure to specific points on the ear to promote healing and relaxation.

2. How does ear reflexology work?

Ear reflexology is based on the idea that the ear is a microsystem of the entire body, and stimulating specific points on the ear can affect corresponding organs and systems in the body. It is believed to help balance the body's energy and promote overall well-being.

3. What conditions can ear reflexology help with?

Ear reflexology is commonly used to help with stress, anxiety, pain management, insomnia, digestive issues, and more. It is often used as a complementary therapy to support overall health and wellness.

4. Is ear reflexology painful?

Ear reflexology is generally not painful, although some people may experience mild discomfort or sensitivity when pressure is applied to certain points on the ear. It should not be painful, and the pressure should be adjusted to your comfort level.

5. How long does a typical ear reflexology session last?

A typical ear reflexology session lasts around 30 to 60 minutes, although this can vary depending on the practitioner and the individual's needs.

6. How many sessions of ear reflexology are needed to see results?

The number of sessions needed can vary depending on the individual and the condition being treated. Some people may experience immediate benefits after one session, while others may require multiple sessions to see significant results.

7. Is ear reflexology safe?

Ear reflexology is generally considered safe when performed by a trained and experienced practitioner. However, it may not be suitable for everyone, especially those with certain medical conditions. It's always best to consult with a healthcare provider before trying any new therapy.

8. Can I do ear reflexology at home?

While it's possible to do some basic ear reflexology techniques at home, it's recommended to seek guidance from a trained practitioner to ensure you are targeting the correct points and using the right techniques.

9. Are there any side effects of ear reflexology?

Side effects of ear reflexology are rare but may include mild discomfort, dizziness, or lightheadedness. It's important to communicate with your practitioner if you experience any adverse effects during or after a session.

10. Is ear reflexology supported by science?

While there is some evidence to suggest that ear reflexology may have benefits for certain conditions, more research is needed to fully understand its effectiveness. Many people find it to be a relaxing and beneficial therapy, but individual experiences can vary.

Expert Answers and Clarifications on Ear Reflexology

1. What is the difference between ear reflexology and foot reflexology?

Ear reflexology and foot reflexology are both based on the principle that specific points on the body correspond to different organs and systems. However, the main difference is the area of the body that is stimulated. Ear reflexology focuses on the ears, while foot reflexology focuses on the feet.

2. Can ear reflexology help with tinnitus?

Some people find that ear reflexology can help reduce the symptoms of tinnitus, such as ringing or buzzing in the ears. However, more research is needed to understand the effectiveness of ear reflexology for tinnitus specifically.

3. Is ear reflexology safe for children?

Ear reflexology can be safe for children when performed by a trained practitioner. It can be a gentle and non-invasive therapy that children may find relaxing. However, it's important to consult with a healthcare provider before trying any new therapy for children.

4. Can ear reflexology help with weight loss?

While ear reflexology is not a direct weight loss treatment, some people believe that stimulating certain points on the ear can help reduce cravings and improve metabolism, which may support weight loss efforts. However, more research is needed to confirm these claims.

5. How often should I receive ear reflexology treatments?

The frequency of ear reflexology treatments can vary depending on the individual and the condition being treated. Some people may benefit from weekly sessions, while others may only need occasional treatments. It's best to consult with a trained practitioner to determine the best treatment plan for you.

6. Can ear reflexology help with sinus congestion?

Some people find that ear reflexology can help reduce sinus congestion and improve sinus drainage. By stimulating certain points on the ear, it's believed to help promote better sinus function. However, individual results may vary.

7. Are there any contraindications for ear reflexology?

Ear reflexology is generally safe for most people, but there are some contraindications to consider. It may not be suitable for individuals with certain medical conditions, such as infections or skin conditions of the ear, or for those who have had recent ear surgery. It's important to consult with a healthcare provider before trying ear reflexology if you have any concerns.

8. Can I combine ear reflexology with other therapies?

Yes, ear reflexology can be combined with other therapies, such as acupuncture, massage, or aromatherapy, to enhance its effects. It's best to discuss your options with a trained practitioner to create a holistic treatment plan that meets your needs.

CHAPTER 12

Recap of Key Points on Ear Reflexology

1.   **Definition:** Ear reflexology, or auriculotherapy, is a form of alternative medicine that involves stimulating specific points on the ear to promote healing and relaxation.

2. **Benefits:** Ear reflexology may help with stress relief, pain management, improved sleep, digestive issues, and more. It is often used as a complementary therapy to support overall health and well-being.

3. Safety: Ear reflexology is generally safe when performed by a trained practitioner. However, it may not be suitable for everyone, especially those with certain medical conditions. It's important to consult with a healthcare provider before trying ear reflexology.

4. Treatment Frequency: The frequency of ear reflexology treatments can vary depending on the individual and the condition being treated. Some people may benefit from weekly sessions, while others may only need occasional treatments.

5. Combination with Other Therapies: Ear reflexology can be combined with other therapies, such as acupuncture, massage, or aromatherapy, to enhance its effects. It's best to discuss your options with a trained practitioner to create a holistic treatment plan.

6. Scientific Evidence: While there is some evidence to suggest that ear reflexology may have benefits for certain conditions, more research is needed to fully understand its effectiveness. Individual experiences with ear reflexology can vary.

7. Contraindications: Ear reflexology may not be suitable for individuals with certain medical conditions, such as infections or skin conditions of the ear, or for those who have had recent ear surgery. It's important to consult with a healthcare provider before trying ear reflexology if you have any concerns.

Encouragement for Further Exploration of Ear Reflexology

If you're intrigued by the potential benefits of ear reflexology, consider exploring this natural therapy further.

Here are some reasons to dive deeper into the world of ear reflexology:

1. Holistic Wellness: Ear reflexology offers a holistic approach to wellness, addressing both physical and mental health. By stimulating specific points on the ear, you can support your body's natural healing processes and promote overall well-being.

2. Self-Care: Learning about ear reflexology can empower you to take control of your health and well-being. You can incorporate simple ear reflexology techniques into your daily routine as a form of self-care and relaxation.

3. Complementary Therapy: Ear reflexology can complement other wellness practices, such as yoga, meditation, and massage. By integrating ear reflexology into your wellness routine, you can enhance the benefits of these practices.

4. Personal Growth: Exploring new therapies like ear reflexology can be a journey of personal growth and self-discovery. You may uncover new ways to support your health and deepen your understanding of your body's natural rhythms.

5. Community and Support: As you delve into the world of ear reflexology, you may find a community of like-minded individuals who share your interest in natural health and wellness. Connecting with others can provide support and encouragement on your wellness journey.

Whether you're seeking relief from stress, pain, or simply looking to enhance your overall well-being, ear reflexology offers a gentle and natural approach to health. Take the time to explore this ancient practice and discover how it can benefit you.

Glossary of Terms in Ear Reflexology

1. **Ear Reflexology:** Also known as auriculotherapy, ear reflexology is a form of alternative medicine that involves stimulating

specific points on the ear to promote healing and relaxation.

2. Auricle: The outer part of the ear, also known as the pinna, where ear reflexology points are located.

3. Auricular Points: Specific points on the ear that correspond to different organs and systems in the body, according to the principles of ear reflexology.

4. Microsystem: The concept that the entire body is represented on a smaller scale within certain areas of the body, such as the ear or the foot, in reflexology.

5. Stimulation: The act of applying pressure, massage, or other techniques to auricular points to elicit a therapeutic response in ear reflexology.

6. Holistic: Considering the whole person, including physical, mental, emotional, and spiritual aspects, in the context of health and wellness.

7. Complementary Therapy: Therapies used alongside conventional medical treatments to support health and well-being, such as ear reflexology.

8. Contraindications: Factors that make a particular treatment or therapy unsafe or inadvisable for an individual, such as certain medical conditions or circumstances.

9. Wellness: A state of overall health and well-being, encompassing physical, mental, emotional, and spiritual aspects.

10. Self-Care: Activities and practices that individuals engage in to promote their own health, well-being, and happiness, such as self-administered ear reflexology techniques.

11. Meridian: In traditional Chinese medicine, meridians are pathways in the body through which vital energy, or qi, flows. Stimulating specific points on the ear is believed to influence the flow of qi along these meridians.

12. Acupressure: A technique similar to acupuncture, acupressure involves applying pressure to specific points on the body, including the ears, to promote relaxation and wellness.

13. Endorphins: Neurotransmitters produced by the body that act as natural painkillers and mood elevators. Ear reflexology is believed to stimulate the release of endorphins, leading to feelings of well-being and pain relief.

14. Reflex Zone: A specific area of the body, such as the ear, that is believed to correspond to other parts of the body. Stimulating reflex zones is thought to have therapeutic effects on the corresponding body parts.

15. Auricular Therapy: Another term for ear reflexology or auriculotherapy, which involves using the ears to diagnose and treat health conditions.

16. Somatotopic Map: A representation of the body on another part of the body, such as the ear.

In ear reflexology, the ear is believed to have a somatotopic map of the entire body, with specific points corresponding to specific organs and systems.

17. Homeostasis: The body's ability to maintain internal balance and stability despite external changes. Ear reflexology is thought to help restore homeostasis by promoting the body's natural healing processes.

18. Trigger Point: A specific point on the body, such as an ear reflexology point, that when stimulated, triggers a therapeutic response in another part of the body.

19. Energy Flow: In traditional Chinese medicine, it is believed that the body's vital energy, or qi, flows through meridians.

Stimulating ear reflexology points is thought to help regulate the flow of energy in the body.

20. Relaxation Response: The body's natural response to relaxation, characterized by reduced heart rate, lowered blood pressure, and a sense of calm. Ear reflexology is believed to elicit this response, promoting relaxation and stress relief.

CONCLUSION

Congratulations on completing your journey through the world of ear reflexology! You have embarked on a path that not only promotes physical healing but also nurtures your mind, body, and spirit. As you conclude this compendium , take a moment to reflect on the knowledge you have gained and the transformations you have experienced.

A Recap of Your Ear Reflexology Journey: Throughout this compendium , you have learned about the anatomy of the ear and how it is mapped for reflexology. You have discovered the principles and techniques of ear reflexology, from basic to advanced, and explored the major and lesser-known reflex points on the ear. You have also gained practical insights into using ear reflexology to address common ailments, integrate it into your daily life, and adapt it for special populations.

Empowering Yourself with Ear Reflexology: By embracing the techniques and principles of ear reflexology, you have taken a proactive step towards enhancing your health and well-being. You have learned that healing is not just about treating symptoms but about addressing the root causes of imbalance in the body. Through ear reflexology, you have discovered a natural and effective way to promote relaxation, reduce stress, manage pain, and improve your overall quality of life.

Continuing Your Ear Reflexology Journey: As you conclude this compendium , remember that your journey with ear reflexology does not end here. Continue to explore and refine your skills, and share your knowledge and experiences with others. Whether you are a seasoned practitioner or a beginner, there is always more to learn and discover in the world of ear reflexology.

Now is the time to take the next step in your ear reflexology journey. Put your knowledge into practice, experiment with different techniques, and explore how ear reflexology can enhance your life. Share your experiences with others and inspire them to embark on their own journey to holistic wellness.

Final Thoughts: As you close this compendium , remember that the power to heal lies within you. By embracing the ancient art of ear reflexology, you have tapped into a source of healing that is as profound as it is natural. May your journey with ear reflexology be a rewarding and transformative one, leading you to a life of balance, harmony, and well-being.

Thank you for joining me on this journey through the world of ear reflexology. May your cars be a gateway to health, happiness, and holistic wellness.

www.ingramcontent.com/pod-product-compliance
Lightning Source LLC
Chambersburg PA
CBHW051607250726

48653CB00004BA/1390